"Invest in your hair,
It's the crown you never take off"

THIS JOURNAL
BELONGS TO

. . . .

There are many reasons for choosing to follow a vegan diet:

Animal welfare: Simply no easier way to help animals than by choosing a plant-based diet over a diet of meat, eggs and dairy 2products.

Climate change:Meat production is one of the biggest causes of pollution.

Health:Being vegan means you are less likely to develop heart disease, cancer, diabetes and high blood pressure.

Weight:vegans are up to 20lbs lighter than their meat eating peers.

Whatever your motivation, there are certain nutrients you must be eating daily to protect the hair growth cycle.

If you have nutrients missing from your diet over a prolonged period, this could result in hair thinning or loss.

How to care for your hair

A good hair care routine will depend on your hair type.
If your hair is **straight** it may get oily more quickly, than if your hair is **curly**, so you may need to wash your hair more often.
If you hair is dyed regularly, it may need more conditioning than natural hair.
Choose a vegan shampoo that is right for your hair type.
Add a conditioner to your routine if your hair feels dry, damaged and lacklustre.

Washing and conditioning your hair:

1 Wet hair with warm water, *(not too hot)*

2 Apply a small amount of shampoo *(about the size of 10 pence piece)*

3 Massage into scalp, working around the back of the head under the occipital bone and into the nape of the neck, pull through mid lengths and ends

4 Rinse really well, do not leave any residue as this can irritate the scalp Repeat if hair is dirty, but usually once is enough.

5 Apply conditioner to mid lengths and ends, comb through, leave for a few minutes

6 Rinse well

7 Wring excess water from hair

8 Pat dry with towel, don't rub as the hair is weakest when wet.

9 Comb through with wide tooth comb, no yanking or tugging remember the hair is weakest when wet.

10 Let the hair dry naturally if possible

If your styling your hair use a heat protector and keep hair driers on a medium temperature and any heated appliance i.e. tongs, straighteners, at 160 – 185 degrees.

Quick Tips:

Use Natural boar bristle brushes as they glide through the hair

Its best to sleep on silk pillowcases.

Daily Must Haves
Week 1

Vegetables

Calcium Rich Foods

Fruits

Vitamins B12 & D Iodine

Nuts & Seeds

Grains

Legumes

6 - 8 Glasses of Water

Recipe Ideas

	Breakfast	Lunch	Dinner	Snacks	Water	Vitamins
Mon						
Tues						
Wed						
Thurs						
Fri						
Sat						
Sun						

Weekly To Do List:

Grocery List:

- ....
- ....
- ....
- ....
- ....
- ....
- ....
- ....
- ....
- ....
- ....
- ....
- ....
- ....
- ....
- ....

Main Tasks:

Exercise Goals:

Reminders:

Reflections on the week:

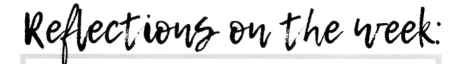

How are you feeling this week?

How was your hair?

"If it doesn't nourish your hair or your soul let it go"

Did you know?

PROTEIN FOODS ACTUALLY BREAK DOWN
INTO 22 NATURALLY OCCURRING
AMINO ACIDS, WHICH ARE KNOWN AS
THE BUILDING BLOCKS OF PROTEIN.

OF THESE,
NINE ARE KNOWN AS ESSENTIAL AMINO
ACIDS, WHICH MEANS WE MUST GET
THEM FROM FOOD, AS THE BODY
CANNOT MAKE THEM ITSELF.

PROTEIN IS ALSO A GOOD SOURCE OF
VITAMINS AND MINERALS SUCH AS ZINC
AND B VITAMINS.

AS A VEGAN, IT'S IMPORTANT THAT ALL
THESE AMINO ACIDS ARE INCLUDED IN
THE DIET TO PROVIDE OPTIMUM
NUTRITION.

Daily Must Haves
Week 2

Vegetables

Calcium Rich Foods

Fruits

Vitamins B12 & D Iodine

Nuts & Seeds

Grains

Legumes

6 - 8 Glasses of Water

Recipe Ideas

Thoughts?

	Breakfast	Lunch	Dinner	Snacks	Water	Vitamins
Mon						
Tues						
Wed						
Thurs						
Fri						
Sat						
Sun						

Weekly To Do List:

Grocery List:

- ....
- ....
- ....
- ....
- ....
- ....
- ....
- ....
- ....
- ....
- ....
- ....
- ....
- ....
- ....
- ....

Main Tasks:

Exercise Goals:

Reminders:

Reflections on the week:

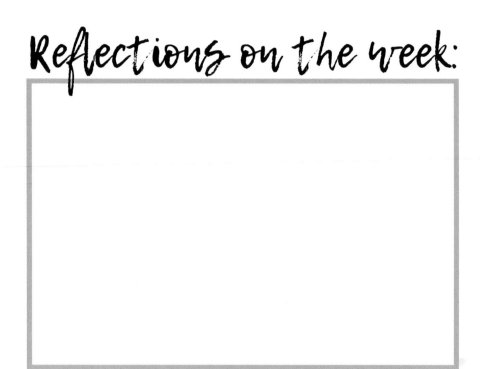

How are you feeling this week?

How was your hair?

Book a hairdresser appointment, keep your locks looking sharp!

Hair Mask
Recipes

The Hulk
Restore amino acids, proteins,
add moisture and sooth:
1 ripe avocado, 2 tbsp olive oil

Monkey Business
Prevents breakage:
1 ripe banana, 2 tbsp olive oil

Blend together, apply to damp hair.
Cover with a shower cap and towel.
Leave for 20-30 mins.
Rinse hair with shampoo.
Apply conditioner.
Allow hair to dry naturally

Daily Must Haves
Week 3

Vegetables

Calcium Rich Foods

Fruits

Vitamins B12 & D Iodine

Nuts & Seeds

Grains

Legumes

6 - 8 Glasses of Water

Recipe Ideas

Thoughts?

	Breakfast	Lunch	Dinner	Snacks	Water	Vitamins
Mon						
Tues						
Wed						
Thurs						
Fri						
Sat						
Sun						

Weekly To Do List:

Grocery List:

- ....
- ....
- ....
- ....
- ....
- ....
- ....
- ....
- ....
- ....
- ....
- ....
- ....
- ....
- ....
- ....

Main Tasks:

Exercise Goals:

Reminders:

Reflections on the week:

How are you feeling this week?

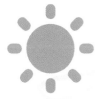 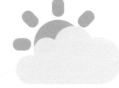

How was your hair?

"Your nicer when you like your hair"

Daily Must Haves
Week 4

Vegetables

Calcium Rich Foods

Fruits

Vitamins B12 & D Iodine

Nuts & Seeds

Grains

Legumes

6 - 8 Glasses of Water

Recipe Ideas

Thoughts?

	Breakfast	Lunch	Dinner	Snacks	Water	Vitamins
Mon						
Tues						
Wed						
Thurs						
Fri						
Sat						
Sun						

Weekly To Do List:

Grocery List:

- ....
- ....
- ....
- ....
- ....
- ....
- ....
- ....
- ....
- ....
- ....
- ....
- ....
- ....
- ....
- ....

Main Tasks:

Exercise Goals:

Reminders:

Reflections on the week:

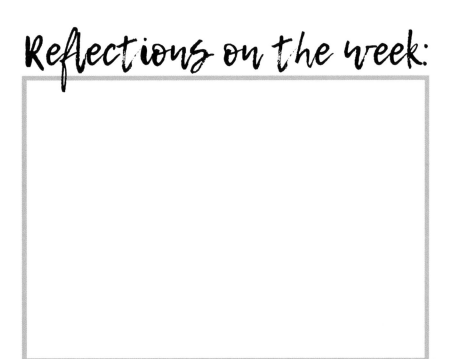

How are you feeling this week?

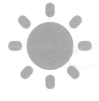

How was your hair?

"Your nicer when you like your hair"

Daily Must Haves
Week 5

Vegetables

Calcium Rich Foods

Fruits

Vitamins B12 & D Iodine

Nuts & Seeds

Grains

Legumes

6 - 8 Glasses of Water

Recipe Ideas

Thoughts?

	Breakfast	Lunch	Dinner	Snacks	Water	Vitamins
Mon						
Tues						
Wed						
Thurs						
Fri						
Sat						
Sun						

Weekly To Do List:

Grocery List:

- ....
- ....
- ....
- ....
- ....
- ....
- ....
- ....
- ....
- ....
- ....
- ....
- ....
- ....
- ....
- ....

Main Tasks:

Exercise Goals:

Reminders:

Reflections on the week:

How are you feeling this week?

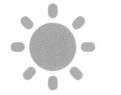 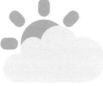

How was your hair?

"Eat, sleep, do hair, repeat"

Daily Must Haves
Week 6

Vegetables

Calcium Rich Foods

Fruits

Vitamins B12 & D Iodine

Nuts & Seeds

Grains

Legumes

6 - 8 Glasses of Water

Recipe Ideas

Thoughts?

	Breakfast	Lunch	Dinner	Snacks	Water	Vitamins
Mon						
Tues						
Wed						
Thurs						
Fri						
Sat						
Sun						

Weekly To Do List:

Grocery List:

- ....
- ....
- ....
- ....
- ....
- ....
- ....
- ....
- ....
- ....
- ....
- ....
- ....
- ....
- ....
- ....

Main Tasks:

Exercise Goals:

Reminders:

Reflections on the week:

How are you feeling this week?

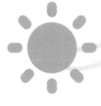 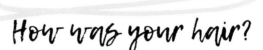

How was your hair?

Book a hairdresser appointment, keep your locks looking sharp.

YOU'RE HALFWAY THERE

You Can Do It

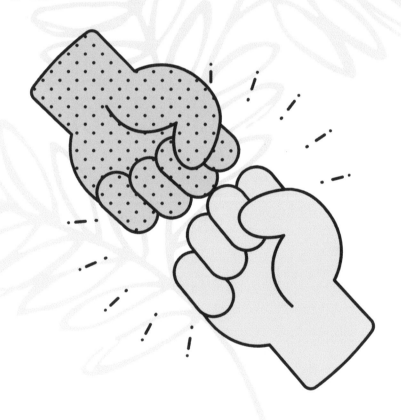

Daily Must Haves
Week 7

Vegetables

Calcium Rich Foods

Fruits

Vitamins B12 & D Iodine

Nuts & Seeds

Grains

Legumes

6 - 8 Glasses of Water

Recipe Ideas

Thoughts?

	Breakfast	Lunch	Dinner	Snacks	Water	Vitamins
Mon						
Tues						
Wed						
Thurs						
Fri						
Sat						
Sun						

Weekly To Do List:

Grocery List:

- ....
- ....
- ....
- ....
- ....
- ....
- ....
- ....
- ....
- ....
- ....
- ....
- ....
- ....
- ....
- ....

Main Tasks:

Exercise Goals:

Reminders:

Reflections on the week:

How are you feeling this week?

How was your hair?

"When your hair is on point, you
can handle anything"

Daily Must Haves
Week 8

Vegetables

Calcium Rich Foods

Fruits

Vitamins B12 & D Iodine

Nuts & Seeds

Grains

Legumes

6 - 8 Glasses of Water

Recipe Ideas

Thoughts?

	Breakfast	Lunch	Dinner	Snacks	Water	Vitamins
Mon						
Tues						
Wed						
Thurs						
Fri						
Sat						
Sun						

Weekly To Do List:

Grocery List:

- ....
- ....
- ....
- ....
- ....
- ....
- ....
- ....
- ....
- ....
- ....
- ....
- ....
- ....
- ....
- ....
- ....

Main Tasks:

Exercise Goals:

Reminders:

Reflections on the week:

How are you feeling this week?

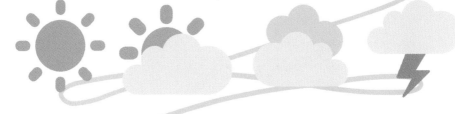

How was your hair?

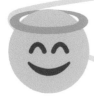

"First do the coffee, then do the hair"

Looking after YOU!

Practice relaxation techniques

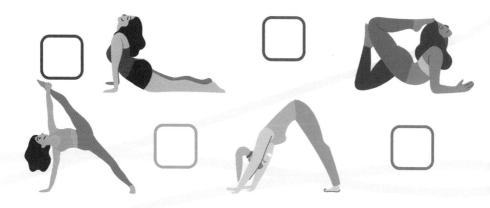

Yoga - There is plenty of free yoga routines on the internet to practice in the comfort of your own home or take up a local class!

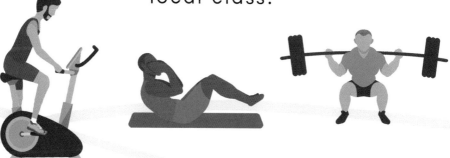

Regular Exercise - A 30 minute daily walk is enough, however doing more doesn't hurt.

Daily Must Haves
Week 9

Vegetables

Calcium Rich Foods

Fruits

Vitamins B12 & D Iodine

Nuts & Seeds

Grains

Legumes

6 - 8 Glasses of Water

Recipe Ideas

Thoughts?

	Breakfast	Lunch	Dinner	Snacks	Water	Vitamins
Mon						
Tues						
Wed						
Thurs						
Fri						
Sat						
Sun						

Weekly To Do List:

Grocery List:

- ....
- ....
- ....
- ....
- ....
- ....
- ....
- ....
- ....
- ....
- ....
- ....
- ....
- ....
- ....
- ....

Main Tasks:

Exercise Goals:

Reminders:

Reflections on the week:

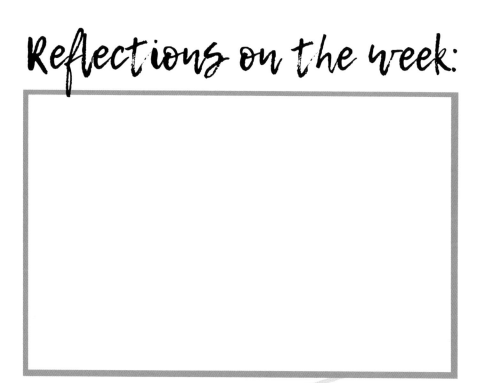

How are you feeling this week?

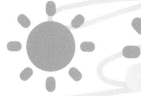

How was your hair?

 "Good hair speaks louder than words"

Daily Must Haves
Week 10

Vegetables

Calcium Rich Foods

Fruits

Vitamins B12 & D Iodine

Nuts & Seeds

Grains

Legumes

6 - 8 Glasses of Water

Recipe Ideas

Thoughts?

	Breakfast	Lunch	Dinner	Snacks	Water	Vitamins
Mon						
Tues						
Wed						
Thurs						
Fri						
Sat						
Sun						

Weekly To Do List:

Main Tasks:

Grocery List:

- ....
- ....
- ....
- ....
- ....
- ....
- ....
- ....
- ....
- ....
- ....
- ....
- ....
- ....
- ....
- ....

Exercise Goals:

Reminders:

Reflections on the week:

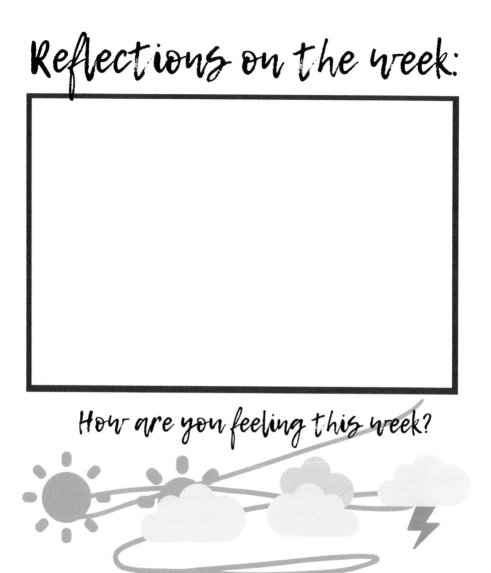

How are you feeling this week?

How was your hair?

"Never give up on your hair journey"

Daily Must Haves
Week 11

Vegetables

Calcium Rich Foods

Fruits

Vitamins B12 & D Iodine

Nuts & Seeds

Grains

Legumes

6 - 8 Glasses of Water

Recipe Ideas

Thoughts?

	Breakfast	Lunch	Dinner	Snacks	Water	Vitamins
Mon						
Tues						
Wed						
Thurs						
Fri						
Sat						
Sun						

Weekly To Do List:

Grocery List:

- ....
- ....
- ....
- ....
- ....
- ....
- ....
- ....
- ....
- ....
- ....
- ....
- ....
- ....
- ....
- ....

Main Tasks:

Exercise Goals:

Reminders:

Reflections on the week:

How are you feeling this week?

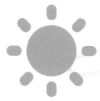  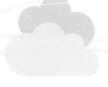

How was your hair?

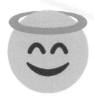

"Good hair doesn't stay home on the weekend"

Foods to Avoid!

Be aware of foods that are high in fat, sugar or heavily processed. These foods can be found in vegan form but should not be relied on as they will not provide the correct nutrition.

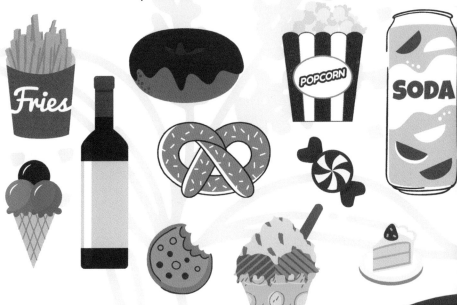

Eat the rainbow

Be sure to eat colourful food. Lots of lovely fruit and veg will ensure the best nutrients for natural hair growth!

Daily Must Haves
Week 12

Vegetables

Calcium Rich Foods

Fruits

Vitamins B12 & D Iodine

Nuts & Seeds

Grains

Legumes

6 - 8 Glasses of Water

Recipe Ideas

Thoughts?

	Breakfast	Lunch	Dinner	Snacks	Water	Vitamins
Mon						
Tues						
Wed						
Thurs						
Fri						
Sat						
Sun						

Weekly To Do List:

Grocery List:

- ....
- ....
- ....
- ....
- ....
- ....
- ....
- ....
- ....
- ....
- ....
- ....
- ....
- ....
- ....
- ....

Main Tasks:

Exercise Goals:

Reminders:

Reflections on the week:

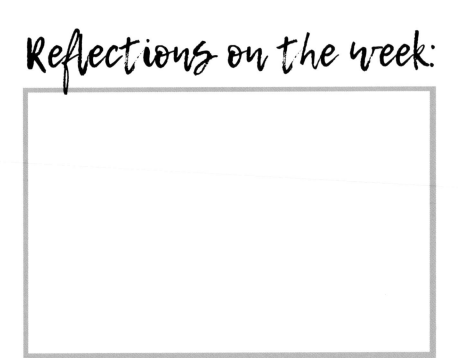

How are you feeling this week?

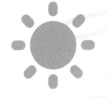 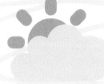 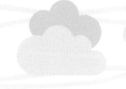

How was your hair?

"Good hair doesn't stay home on the weekend"

Notes

....
....
....
....
....
....
....
....
....
....
....
....
....
....
....
....
....
....
....
....
....
....
....
....
....

Congratulations

YOU'VE DONE IT

In order to maintain your new found locks,
be sure to follow the advice given in your journal!

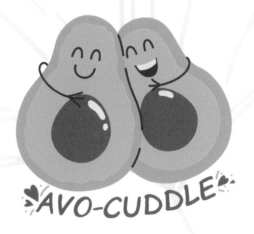

Should you want to know more or get yourself a little support, why not follow us on social media?

 facebook.com/hlcclondon

 @LondonHLCC

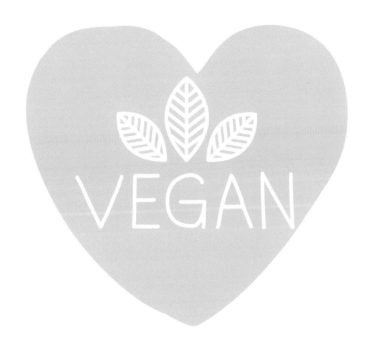

 Designed by Jessica Harris

Printed in Great Britain
by Amazon